AF223821

PERFECT ESSENTIAL OILS

WHAT YOU WISH YOU KNEW ABOUT ESSENTIAL OILS

JAMIE J.

CONTENTS

©Copyright 2022 – All rights reserved by Jamie J.

The content of this book may not be reproduced, duplicated, or transmitted without direct written permission from the author or publisher.

ISBN-978-1-63970-132-2

Legal Notice:

This book is copyright protected. This is only for personal use. You cannot amend, distribute, sell, use, quote, or paraphrase any part of the content within this book without the consent of the author or publisher.

Disclaimer notice:

Please note the information contained within this document is for educational and entertainment purposes only.

Every attempt has been made to provide accurate, up-to-date, and reliable complete information.

No warranties of any kind are expressed or implied. Readers acknowledge that the author is not engaging in the rendering of legal, financial, medical or professional advice. The content of this book has been derived from various sources. Please consult a licensed professional before attempting any techniques outlined in this book.

By reading this document, the reader agrees that under no circumstances is the author responsible for any losses, direct or indirect, which are incurred as a result of the use of the information contained within this document, including, but not limited to, -errors, omissions, or inaccuracies.

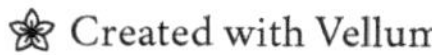 Created with Vellum

INTRODUCTION

Essential Oils.

A massage is a common form of treating the body, therapeutically or otherwise, using a body part to enhance or relax other body parts. You see this in all cultures and regions of the world.

The word means to 'knead' whether it be the French word massage, the Arabic 'massa', or even the Greek 'masso'.

People have often wondered how a relaxing and comforting treatment cures ailments of the body and mind. Ancient Ayurvedic texts explain toxins accumulate daily in the issues, and a massage dissolves them and slowly removes them from the system.

Ayurveda also goes on and recommends 'Abhyanga' or oil massage as part of everyday life. The texts go on and list out the benefits. Some of them are:

It is nourishing to the body

Reduces fatigue

Stimulates relaxed and deep sleep

Provides stamina

Improves the complexion and luster of the skin

Detoxifies

Improves longevity

Increased circulation to the nerve endings

Toning of the whole muscle structure

Soothes the nerves

Lubricates joints

Improves mental alertness

These are some of the benefits that are seen among people who indulge in a massage daily.

Massages serve many purposes, from treating an ailing part of the body to enhancing the reflexes to a warm relaxing, or sensual one. It is usually done by using both hands, but nowadays, sensual massages involve body o body massage.

When a massage is applied, there are many things to consider: the ambiance, the pressure used, the body condition, and even the medium used. We will be mainly discussing the medium here in this book as it is of utmost importance.

Most massages are done using base oils. These are good as they nourish the skin and act as medicine for most skin ailments. The most popular ones are Jojoba, Wheat Germ, and Olive oil. These are added to any primary oil to improve its medicinal value.

Essential oils differ from Base oils as the former are derived from extracting concentrated essences from seeds, fruit, or other plant sources. As a result, these double in their therapeutic value also.

WHAT IS AROMATHERAPY?

Aromatherapy is a type of massage that uses Essential Oils sourced from unique plants. This type of massage is used for two purposes: 1) enhance the mood and 2) get rid of or reduce pain.

Practitioners of Aromatherapy are called Aromatherapists, and they use Essential Oils in a diluted form as most of the Essential Oils are concentrated and may be harmful to the body. The Oils are diluted with other Natural Oils called Base or Carrier Oils.

A Therapist usually blends oils to a maximum of five to get the desired effect on the body. For example, a massage for a sprain or cramp may use Eucalyptus oil, while a relaxing massage uses Lavender.

Aromatherapy Oils are also seen used widely in sensual massages as many of the Essential Oils have Aphrodisiacal effects.

. . .

Many of the Aromatherapy Oils from trusted blenders can be used in baths or a massage session at home. As the Essential oils are pure, they often tend to be volatile, so care should be given while storing them for later use. Some Essential Oils have a longer shelf life, and these are the ones that you should select if you plan to keep them for later use.

Essential Oils are sourced from plants and trees or parts of them like the kernel, flower, or bark, and the oils must be used with advice from a recommended practitioner as it may be allergic to some skin types.

Aromatherapy is often confused with terms like scented or perfumed oils. The latter oils are blended with chemicals and should never be used. A room that is scented and used for massage also does not make it an Aromatherapy session. Aromatherapy uses Essential Oils, and that is the only thumb rule.

A Brief History on aromatherapy

The use of herbs ad plant derived oils for the benefit of massage has been popular in countries like India, China, and Italy from ancient times. It was not until 1937 when Rene Maurice Gattefose, the French practitioner, witnessed the use of Lavender Oil on skin burns and used the term Aromatherapy.

Aromatherapy is very popular now on a worldwide level and is often used in Alternative and Holistic treatments. In Europe and

North America, there are a lot of spas that offer Aromatherapy for multiple benefits.

Why is Aromatherapy Effective?

Aromatherapy uses Essential Oils, these are natural and so does not have side effects that are usually associated with medicines. These plant derived oils can stimulate and cure almost all organs and parts of the body. They also have profound Pharmacological benefits too and are anti-bacterial, detoxifying and stimulating to name a few benefits.

Essential Oils stimulate the Limbic System that is responsible for the emotions and controls the glands to release hormones. Inhaling the molecules present in these oils can stimulate the Pituitary and Hypothalamus and reduce stress, boost memory and maintain hormonal balance. They also help in alleviating nasal congestion and bring about an immediate effect on the moods and balance on a physiological level.

As a rule:

Lavender, Geranium and Chamomile oils have a calming effect.

Rosemary oil is good for energizing and cleaning.

Ylang Ylang, Neroli, Rose, and Clary Sage oils have an uplifting effect.

. . .

Pine Tree oils and Eucalyptus are good to remove congestions and pain.

USES OF ESSENTIAL OILS

Therapeutic and medicinal uses

As mentioned earlier, massages are done for many healthy treatments of the body. This doesn't make it a treatment just for the ailing, it can be done on a healthy body also. But massages are mainly done with a therapeutic aim.

Research has proved that massages have a lot of benefits which include relief from pain and even reduced stress levels and, pressure, heart rate, and anxiety.

Even though massages are done as a relaxer or as a great foreplay technique, it still instills a feel of energy and health to the body. Using oils is highly recommended by countries like India and China, where this has been practice for many centuries. It is also important to know what type of oils or gels (which is popular now as it is easier to wash off but not recommended) to use when applying a massage.

. . .

Understanding massage oils

Well, the introduction may have been a little daunting to the novice, but it's not all that geeky. In fact, after you read this book, you will be up and ready to give your first massage with confidence.

The basic purpose of massage oils is to act as a medium. What the medium does is to act as a layer over the skin and assist in a smooth movement all around it. Massage involves a smooth and unbroken movement throughout the session. The oils also reduces friction and the heat developed by it.

There is also a secondary level of benefit like nourishing the body, especially the skin and providing as a carrier in Aromatherapy! But let's not complicate things!

The best thing about oils is that it is completely natural. All we have to do now is to compare oils on the following criteria:

Spread of the oil: There are many oils in the market, some are of a baby oil consistency while the more medicinal are thick and a bit sticky. When starting out on massages, it is best to go for one widespread over the body.

Absorption: A good massage involves the maximum touch. If the oil is too slow to be absorbed by the skin, the pleasure derived can be lost as the body may be too slippery and you have to massage more than what is usually required.

Aroma: All oils smell different. Another person may not like an oil smell that you like in particular. When selecting an oil, go for one with a light scent or one scented naturally. The most popular scents being lime and orange. Just ensure that the oils are scented naturally, or you can do so by lightly warming the oil with dried rinds of lime or orange added to it.

As a rule of thumb, the best selection is a cold pressed extra virgin. These oils are known for retaining all the natural nutrients and the purity.

Massage is now popular among almost all people, and the market is just booming with newer scents and newer price tags attached. When planning to buy oil for massage, you need to have a budget in mind. This s when you need to go for Essential Oils.

UNDERSTANDING MASSAGE OILS

Most Popular essential oils

The most used Essential Oils are:

Sunflower Oil: This is the most cost-effective oil in the market. It has a considerably decent spread and a nourishing effect on the skin. The only drawback is that it may become a bit sticky and most of the brands come heat pressed, hence having a short shelf life.

Almond Oil: This is the most popular one, especially the sweet almond oil. All brands are reasonably priced, and the oil has a good spread, better absorption, and is totally non greasy. It also has a light scent is very nourishing for the skin.

. . .

Grape Seed Oil: This is second in the list and has a good absorption value clinging on to the non-greasy oils. It is worth the buy but a bit pricier than almond oil.

The list is unending, so we have compiled a list of Essential/Aromatherapy oils based on their therapeutic effects and popularity

Lavender Oil: Is very popular owing to its scent that is pleasing to all and due to its calming effects. It calms the mind and rids of anxiety and is among the oils that can be applied directly on the skin and even on stings and burns. It eases the pain and has antiseptic properties.

Ylang Ylang: Is a must have Essential Oil. It suits all skin types, oily or dry and also cures it on regular application. It has a sedating property and soothes the nervous system and induces sleep when massaged with it. It also helps in the circulation of blood and helps in producing endorphins which reduce body pains.

Tea Tree Oil: This also can be applied directly to cuts and stings as it has anti-inflammatory and antiseptic properties. It is an effective oil in curing and blemishes of the skin or damage to it, for that matter, and soothes the respiratory system.

Eucalyptus Oil: This has long been known for its medicinal value. It is good in soothing body pains related to cramps and sprains. It also heals ad prevents scar blemishes and tissues. It is also a popular bath oil as it soothes congested air passages and is stimulating to the senses.

. . .

Though these sum up most of the popular oils, there are others also which are in the market and is used for massage. We will take a quick glance at these also.

As most of the oils used for massages are natural, you will quite surely find them in local food stores. But if you plan to visit a body shop or a spa store, you can buy blended oils that contain more than one of the oils.

While listing out other oils, we can go a bit further on the properties of the oil.

Apricot Kernel Oil: This oil is an abundant source of Vitamin E, an essential vitamin for skin care. It has a good enough shelf life. The texture and color is similar to that of Sweet Almond oil and is on the non-greasy side. Though this is costlier than its counterpart, Apricot Kernel Oil can be substituted for Sweet Almond Oil if you have an allergy to nuts.

Jojoba Oil: Though they call it oil, it is a wax derived from the Jojoba seed. Jojoba oil has antibacterial values, and the wax is like skin sebum. Jojoba oil has a very extensive shelf life and can be stored if you usually use other oils for massage. Jojoba does not cause skin irritation and can be used on all skin types. It is fast-absorbing, and you need to use more of it for or blend it with other oils. Again, this is a bit pricy.

Coconut Oil (Fractionated): Coconut oil has a lot of good properties, but when it comes to being used as a massage oil, it is better to go for Fractionated ones. Fractionated oils are blended oils that contain just a fraction of the oil. Coconut oil is naturally a bit greasy. Fractionated Coconut Oils are on the economic side and resemble Sweet Almond Oil. It has a durable shelf life that lasts long. This oil also does not stain sheets like most of the massage oils.

Avocado Oil: Avocado oil has a dark green color and can add a bit of that ambiance if you have a collection of oils. It is also thick and usually can be blended with lighter oils to add body to them. It is doubly pricy than the popular Sweet Almond Oil, and if you are prone to latex irritation, you should stay away from this.

Cocoa Butter Oil: Cocoa Butter is the best for skincare, and tall admire the rich flavor. It has a very thick consistency and is usually mixed with lighter oils. Some people apply it without diluting when smaller areas of the body are massaged.

Kukui Oil: Yes, you guessed that right! Kukui Oil is a native of the Hawaiian Islands and is suitable for all skin types. It is also good at soothing sunburnt skin.

Olive Oil: Though popular as a food oil, Olive Oil is used widely in massage parlors. It is thick and has a distinctive flavor, and for these reasons, it is usually blended with other oils.

Sesame Seed Oil: Sesame Seed Oil is a must have in Ayurveda and is advised for daily use. It has detoxifying properties and is good for skin ailments, bloating and even constipation. The oil has a heavy aroma and is usually mixed with other aromatic oils.

· · ·

Shea Butter: Shea Butter is an oil extracted from the Shea tree which is found in Africa. It is called butter as it has a very thick body and is usually blended with other oils as it leaves the skin rather greasy.

Wheat Germ: This is a rich source of Vitamin E and owing to its rather thick consistency. It is usually mixed rather than used by itself.

Argan Oil: Though not very popular, Argan Oil extracted from the Argania Spinosa tree, a native of the Moroccan lands, is a rich source of Vitamin E and other essential fatty acids. It can also be consumed as a medicine. It is usually said to reverse the effects of ageing and has a beneficial impact on the hair and nails.

Jasmine Oil: This is not a common oil in massage parlors but widely used in sensual massages. Jasmine is a natural aphrodisiac and the fumes affect the emotion controlling part of the body called the Limbic System. It is also good in reducing stress and stress related symptoms.

Rose Oil: This is a very popular oil when it comes to Aroma Therapy. This also affects the Limbic System when applied on the skin or by just inhaling it. Just like Jasmine oil, it is used to treat Menstrual and Menopausal troubles.

Rosemary Oil: Rosemary is a Mediterranean herb and the oil derived from it has many beneficial values. It is thought to have medicinal values for the brain and reduces stress and also helps in recovering patients suffering from Alzheimer's.

. . .

Lemon Oil: This is a very refreshing oil and helps stimulate the brain and prevent Alzheimer's. It is also widely used in cutting weight and those unwanted fat deposits.

Bergamot Oil: This is extracted from a type of citrus fruit and has all the benefits of Lemon oil and a plus benefit as a cure for ringworms.

Helichrysum Oil: This is an oil derived from a flower of the Sunflower family. This has been long used in Aromatherapy and has many health benefits. It has antifungal and antibacterial effects and is a cure for many skin diseases like acne, burns, and insect bites. It is also sometimes used to treat arthritis. It also has strong detoxing effects and also helps in anti-aging by boosting the Immune System.

Patchouli Oil: This oil comes from the tropics and is derived from the leaves of the Patchouli or the Pogostemon cablin herb. You might have seen it listed in the ingredients of skincare creams. If inhaled or applied to the skin, this oil has many benefits as it stimulates the Limbic System. Like most oils that offer the same effect, this oil also reduces stress and stress related symptoms. It is also known to cure congestions of the nasal tract.

Geranium Oil: Is derived from the geranium plant or the Pelargonium graveolens. It is a rich source of Geraniol and Citronellol, which are plant compounds that boost health. Inhaling or applying this oil has a lot of beneficial effects. It has anti-bacterial and anti-fungal properties. This oil can be administered orally and is shown to have detox effects. This also has been used widely as a cure for insomnia.

Do it yourself tips

A Word of Caution:
Most Essential Oils come in a concentrated level, and even minimal amounts can irritate the skin. However, too much of it can cause an aver dose and can burn the skin.

Essential Oils are not recommended for usage near the eyes, ears, or nose. Never take crucial Oil, even in small quantities, internally.

Some oils like Citrus Oil and Grapefruit Oil can be harmful to your skin if applied and exposed to sunlight.

Always go for a patch test before trying out any Essential oil. Dabbing a small amount on your arm and testing the reaction is always a good thing to do.

Use an area with a good flow of air if you plan to make your Essential Oil blends.

Consulting a qualified practitioner is highly advised if you have any health conditions or allergies to certain foods and oils.

· · ·

Here are some things to keep in mind when buying Essential Oils:

We have already mentioned that Essential Oils are concentrated and come in a variety of aromas. Hold the bottle about 5 inches from your nose when sniffing, as if the bottle is too close it may cause irritation and a burning sensation to your air passage.

Don't take a marathon sniffing trial. Instead, take frequent breaks and take a whiff of fresh air. Essential oils have solid fumes, and too much may make you giddy.

If a brand sells all its Essential Oils at the same price tag, then it is a litmus test as to the quality of the Oil. This is because different oils have different prices according to the availability and cost of the raw material. Usually, the same price on all oils is a telltale sign that it is an abundant synthetic material.

Buy Oils from brands that name the ingredients in their English name and scientific name. They should also mention the method used for extraction and the country from which it comes.

Only buy oils that list it as 100%. Any oils labelled under perfumed or fragrant are mixed with chemicals.

Never buy Essential Oils that come in plastic or clear bottles. Deep Blue and Amber bottles should be preferred as they let in limited light. In addition, oils lose their value if exposed to sunlight. This is also a tip that you should have in mind when storing your oils.

How to Make Essential Oils:

If it is an Essential Oil that you want to make, you need to have a dark blue or amber bottle that can hold 10 ml. of Oil. This should never be applied as such but blended with other oils.

A massage-ready Oil can be made and stored in a 125 ml dispenser of the colors mentioned above. If you plan to make one that you may frequently use, then a bigger bottle can be used, but you should take special care about the Oil's shelf life.

Relaxing oil blend

Ingredients:

1. Lavender Oil
2. Chamomile Oil
3. Sandalwood Oil
4. Ylang Ylang Oil
5. Regular Massage Oil

All the oils mentioned above are Essential Oils, and the last one i.e., Regular Massage oil, is optional.

For a 10 ml dispenser of Blended Oil, use:

. . .

1 tsp. and 20 drops of ingredient a
    30 drops of ingredients b and c
    20 drops ingredient d
    To make desired Massage Oil (4 fl. oz)
    25 drops of ingredient a
    6 drops of ingredients b and c
    5 drops of ingredient d

Top up with a massage oil of your choice.

Once you have made your blends, sure to label them appropriately. This is a must as some people are allergic to some oils.

Chamomile oils come in different names. The Roman one is a muscle relaxant, whereas its German counterpart decreases inflammation.

ESSENTIAL OIL BLEND (SORE MUSCLES)
    Essential Oil Blend (Sore Muscles):
    Ingredients:

1. Roman Chamomile Oil
2. Peppermint Oil
3. Lavender Oil
4. Clary Sage Oil
5. Regular Massage Oil

For a 125 ml dispenser, you will need:
    14 drops of ingredients a and c

8 drops ingredient c

4 drops of ingredient d

After mixing the ingredients, top it up with regular massage oil.

The benefits of massages are many, and oil massage, especially one that uses Essential Oils, should be done daily and become a lifestyle.

Though Aromatherapy is booming today, you should give considerable attention to the oils they use and not get confused with marketing terms like Perfumed and Fragrance oil massages as they may use chemicals in oils.

The End.

Did you like this book? Then you'll LOVE Aromatherapy and Essential Oils: The Ultimate Guide to Essential Oils for Healing and Essential Oils Recipes

As you will see in this book, Aromatherapy, the art, and science of using essential oils for a purpose that will give a better quality of life, has been around since ancient times in several parts of the globe but is still a favorite subject among scientific studies and research. It's not just that almost magical scents of these oils that perked our senses and insistence for truth and knowledge, which makes the subject of tempting aromatherapy medical-wise. But the various properties that are potent enough to provide us with confidence to seek the natural way of preventing or treating disease—healing our scarred physical, mental, and emotional systems, and strengthening our health and longevity in general.

Click here to start reading Aromatherapy and Essential Oils NOW!

Aromatherapy and Essential Oils: The Ultimate Guide to Essential Oils for Healing and Essential Oils Recipes

https://books2read.com/u/mqwqO6

Click here to start reading Aromatherapy and Essential Oils NOW!

Aromatherapy and Essential Oils: The Ultimate Guide to Essential Oils for Healing and Essential Oils Recipes

https://books2read.com/u/mqwqO6

———

History of Aromatherapy

What You Need to Know about Essential Oils' Beginnings

The exact beginning of Aromatherapy is impossible to determine. Historians can only logically point to the possibility that Aromatherapy is an accident in its discovery just after the discovery of fire. On the other hand, earth and man probably witnessed the birth of Aromatherapy when the latter became more adept in making fire out of dry wood, leaves, and any of Mother Nature's flammable materials. In one of his amateurish pyrotechnics, he might have used cedar or cypress as firewood or burned tree saps or resin, from which a unique, fragrant scent arose. However, it is very similar to a type of Aromatherapy we now referred to as incense.

Prehistorically. A stroke of luck only discovered incense – it doesn't serve any purpose. However, the Neolithic Era and the Age of Ancient Civilizations have seen the great importance of scent in everyday life and culture and used it for various purposes, including religious ceremonies, relaxation, and healing.

From 7000 – 4000 BC, two other vital pieces of knowledge in Aromatherapy still exist today are mixing plant parts with heated animal fats to produce a scented fat containing the plant's unique aromatics, protective elements, etc. healing and energizing properties. This practice is the origin of modern massage oil and lotion. Another is the creation of aromatic water from plant oils and alcohol mixed in water. Such substance for consumption as a medicinal tonic during ancient times, but its form, properties, and concoction methods are akin to those of present-day perfumes.

The history of Aromatherapy comes from unearthed Egyptian stone tablets. For example, one mural adorning Queen Hatshepsut's temple walls portrays sacks of frankincense traded from Pwenet or the historical Land of Punt. Even Imhotep, an Egyptian, a doctor, and priest credited as the grandfather of Aromatherapy, used these methods. Archaeologists also reported that the tomb of Tutankhamen filled the air with scents of spikenard and myrrh when opened.

These pieces of evidence show that the Egyptians were far more advanced and established with the use of essential oils. Aromatherapy was an indispensable part of their lives. It was not limited to royalties and the members of high society – even commoners could use it. Frankincense such as myrrh, jasmine, cassia oils, and cedarwood for religious ceremonies. Or rituals and mummification, and as an alternative for healing, and toiletries. Fragrant oils were also added to the bath to improve the beauty, refresh the mind, and lift the moods, or applied to the body as perfume and protection against the harsh sun and climate.

Frankincense fragrances. Such as myrrh and other oils from saffron, spikenard, lilies, and cinnamon herbs. They lie depicted in the Old Testament, particularly in Isaiah and Solomon's song. The Hebrews brought with them the practice of using plant and animal oils and essences from the Egyptians when they returned to Israel after the Exodus. The Greeks obtained knowledge from the Egyptians, and both civilizations considered the fragrant plant essences as gods' gifts to men. Romans, in turn, learned it from the Greeks. Perfumes were like a fashion trend in the Roman Empire. Simultaneously, China learned of the art through trade with other civilizations.

Ancients used Aromatherapy for therapeutic purposes known as Ayurveda, traditionally practiced in India for at least 3,000 years. Ancient Hindu texts suggested that sandalwood, myrrh, ginger, rose, and coriander in use as fragrances during rituals. India is the birthplace of Buddhism and Hinduism. Both religions knew incense to honor gods and drive away demons and evil spirits.

Aromatherapy reached the lands of Europe following the return of Crusaders who traveled to the Holy Land. It became a craft and livelihood throughout the Middle Ages, particularly in Grasse, France, a city tagged as the world's perfume capital. Therefore, it's no surprise that the person who prominently worked to reintroduce and finally stabilize the health and medical importance of Aromatherapy in the Modern era is a French "essential oil" connoisseur.

Rene Maurice Gattefosse, a cosmetologist and chemist, studied essential oils' antibiotic and disinfecting properties for more than 50 years. He began testing his theories in 1936 after accidentally burning his arm and personally witnessing the power of lavender oil to lessen the pain of his burns and cure them quickly. As a result, he was the one who first used the term "aromatherapy," which is Aromatherapy in French.

Other experts have followed Gattefosse's theories and work hitherto. Gattefosse's colleague Godissart introduced Aromatherapy in the US as a treatment of severe diseases. In the 1950s, French biochemist Marguerite Maury suggested that the body best absorbed essential oils through massage. Together with Micheline Arcier, she started several European clinics that offered personally concocted blends to treat each patient's specific illness.

After taking a down-time due to the rise to fame of synthetic drugs in the field of medicine, Aromatherapy re-entered the mainstream as a natural way of curing disease. As of present, it is one of the most sought-after alternatives to disease treatment and an indispensable element in areas of beauty, cosmetics, and stress relief.

HOW AROMATHERAPY AND ESSENTIAL OILS WORK THEIR MAGIC

Essential oils possess properties that give potent reactions to the body in physical, mental, and even spiritual aspects. They are powerful energy and immune system stimulants and relaxants with antiseptic, analgesic, and antidepressant properties. Due to these properties, essential oils are now an indispensable item in healing practices, particularly in treating physical wounds, pains, skin infections, and even psychological illnesses such as depression and insomnia. Essential oils can reestablish the balance in hormones and body energies (chakras) at a cellular level. They can also significantly relieve stress and personal issues like low self-esteem, grief, and low moods.

The common idea in modern medicine is 1 compound, say aspirin, equals one batch of properties that will serve the compound's healing purpose. Essential oil, on the other hand, is a mixture of different combinations with unique sets of properties. Yet despite this diversity of compounds in a single substance, essential oil and its various therapeutic effects can work synergistically and supply what the body needs from it. But how can these oils work their magic, technically speaking?

Essential oils can naturally increase oxygen amounts in the air in a closed and narrow space. In a layman's chemistry version, essential oils boost the ozone and negative ions in a given atmosphere, inhibiting bacterial growth and the foul odors from microbial build-ups. They can also get easily attracted to chemical bonds of toxic chemicals present in the air, destroying them and making them safe and breathable. Essential oils remove poisonous substances from the body in the same way, i.e., organically binding with toxins and forming new substances. The body can easily flush the substances out of the body.

Essential oils can successfully get inside us through our olfactory, digestive and integumentary (skin) systems. Probably the oldest and most well-known medium through which essential oils combine to give the desired effects to the body is the olfactory system. Particularly the nose since, as already mentioned, it's highly probable (and logical) that Aromatherapy was first discovered in the form of incense – a fragrant, relaxing scent coming from a burning botanical source. In the eventual rise of civilizations and the formation of cities, cultures, and technologies, essential oils became revered in areas of health and beauty, utilized not only as burned incenses but also as ingestible solutions and topical salves.

Integumentary System

The human skin is the biggest organ that acts as the body's protection against damaging agents from the outside. It contains millions of openings where hair protrudes – a system that adds up to its natural permeability. Like hormone replacement creams and nicotine patches, these oils blend into the skin. The absorption and effects at the cellular level can be significantly hastened, usually within 20 minutes, thru massaging or rubbing. The heat and controlled movements in the area increase blood and oxygen circulation, enhancing the absorption of essential oils.

According to some studies, the absorption rate is faster in

body areas where the sweat glands and hair follicles concentrate, specifically in the genitalia, palms, soles of the feet, head, and armpits.

Olfactory System

The olfactory system is the group of organs or cells that work together to carry out the functions and processes contributing to or related to the sense and perception of scent. This system's most utilized and probably official member is the nose and its parts, though the mouth can transport these scents.

When we inhale through the nose or mouth, airborne molecules possessing odors travel through the opening and interact with olfactory organs that simultaneously transport signals to the brain. The brain has several receptor sites, but the location of interest is the limbic system, also known as the "emotional brain." The limbic system works with the other brain parts that regulate heart rate, breathing, hormone balance, and blood pressure.

This connection is the main reason why electrochemical messages received by the limbic system can significantly trigger emotions and memories. On the outside, we usually associate smells with specific events in our lives. The trigger and release of sedating or stimulating neurochemicals via the use of essential oils take advantage of this process, providing such profound influence on our physiological and psychological systems and functions.

. . .

The odor molecules don't just stop in the brain but travel to the lungs and parts of the respiratory system. Therefore, it is safe to say that the effects of essential oils can reach other parts of the body through several pathways. For example, inhaling peppermint is widely practiced reducing dizziness and fatigue, and eucalyptus is great for treating coughs and sore throat.

Digestive System

Another main pathway through which essential oils enter the body is via ingestion or swallowing. Drinking concocted essential oils was practiced since the glorious days of the Egyptian, Greek, and Roman civilizations.

However, the public is discouraged by experts from ingesting essential oils due to the limitations of studies and experiments in knowledge regarding its safety if swallowed directly in concentrated amounts. Some studies declare that some essential oils can damage the digestive system, particularly if denatured by gastric processes. Others claim that these plant oils can significantly toxically eat significant organs like the liver and kidneys. In addition, doctors discourage ingestion of essential oils for patients who regularly intake meds for their specific illnesses because the compounds in these oils can potentially weaken or damage such drugs' effectiveness or combine with the chemicals in drugs to produce a fatal product. As of present, there are few groups of people who believe in the efficacy of essential oil application through ingestion, albeit practiced only under the strict guidance of expert physicians or pharmacists.

End of Sneal Peek

Click here to start reading Aromatherapy and Essential Oils NOW!

Aromatherapy and Essential Oils: The Ultimate Guide to Essential Oils for Healing and Essential Oils Recipes

https://books2read.com/u/mqwqO6

www.ingramcontent.com/pod-product-compliance
Lightning Source LLC
Chambersburg PA
CBHW061648050726
47598CB00004B/1503